Natural Skin Care

How To Look Younger Cure Acne And Get Mistaken For A College Student - *With Anti Aging Foods And Natural Skin Care*

Table of Contents

Contents

Copyright © 2015 by Fia Furmont

Introduction

Have you ever looked in the mirror and thought, what happened to my skin? I know that I did. When I was younger I never had a problem with my skin. It was always clear and smooth. Even when I was a teenager I didn't have to big of a problem with acne. But it seemed like as I started to get older everything started to change. Suddenly my skin just wasn't as healthy and it just didn't look as good. I started looking older before I knew it and I *hated* it.

I tried just about everything I could think of to get my skin looking great again. To be perfectly honest I never thought much about being 'all natural' before. So I tried pretty much every product available looking to get my skin clearer before I finally arrived at this regimen which provides me (and can provide you) with clearer, healthier skin without compromising on natural ingredients.

I am now a believer that the natural way is the way to go if you're looking to keep your skin looking great. I've seen firsthand what it can actually do and how much improvement it really makes and that's what I'm going to talk about throughout this book, the natural remedy.

Chapter 1: The Overlooked Holy Grail of Looking Younger

I was never a big meat person to begin with and I actually would avoid eating meat not because I was a vegetarian but because I just didn't care for the taste. Unfortunately, since I wasn't a vegetarian, I also wasn't eating a whole lot of fruits and vegetables. What I've found is something that basically everyone already knows, fruits and vegetables contain a lot of vitamins and minerals.

All those vitamins and minerals are great for every single part of your body and definitely for your skin. The problem is most people just don't think about eating fruit and vegetables. Every now and then they sound good so you buy some grapes or a bag of oranges or apples. But then, if you're like my family, they end up going to waste because you completely forget that they are there. (Or you refuse to buy them in the first place because you know that's what's going to happen.)

A lot of people really don't think about how important these things are for your overall health either. Sure you've been told by people all your life but that doesn't mean you're actually listening, paying attention or really concerned. Most people (myself included) assume that 'bad things just don't happen to me.' They figure that aging, wrinkles, dark spots, sagging skin and even cancer just aren't going to happen to them because … well none of us really knows *why*.

The truth of the matter is that these things happen to anyone. When you eat fruits and vegetables and get all the vitamins that are contained inside of them you're reducing the risk of developing these problems. Of course nothing can guarantee that you won't experience the signs of aging but you can definitely cut down on your risk if you work hard to eat foods that contain these ingredients. For a moment we're going to get technical and give you some of the information you need to motivate you to include the foods in your daily diet.

Vitamin C – Reduces the risk of skin cancer and sunburn caused by prolonged exposure to the sun. This vitamin also reduces the risk of damage to the DNA found in skin cells which means your cells (and your skin) are better capable of repairing damage. This vitamin also helps cut back on the damage you suffer from free radicals which can cause damage to collagen and elastin in your skin (causing you to develop wrinkles). This vitamin is found in bell peppers, broccoli, cauliflower, citrus fruit and leafy greens.

Vitamin E – Similar to Vitamin C in many ways, Vitamin E also reduces your risk of damage to DNA in skin cells, reduces the harmful effects of free radicals on the skin and even reduces the damage caused by sun exposure. It also assists with cutting down on photo damage, wrinkles and the texture of your skin. This vitamin is in spinach and asparagus as well as other healthy foods like nuts, seeds and olives.

Vitamin A – Lack of Vitamin A causes dry, flaky skin. What it does is help soften your skin and repair it whenever you experience damage (such as cuts or scrapes). Without enough Vitamin A you start to get dry skin. It can also cause wrinkles, acne breakouts, and psoriasis (or at least worse effects from any of these. Luckily, Vitamin A is easy to find. It's in just about anything you eat and especially in almost all fruits and vegetables.

Vitamin K – This vitamin can actually be used topically for the best effects on your skin, which means you don't need to eat a lot of fruits and vegetables that have it (at least not for skin benefits). When you do put it on your skin however it can actually remove signs of dark circles under your eyes, definitely something that makes you look older.

Vitamin B Complex – These are possibly the most important vitamins to your skin. One of them, biotin, is responsible for skin, nail and hair cells and without it, your will start to suffer. In fact, too little biotin can result in dermatitis and hair loss. This vitamin can perform near miracles when you use it topically too because it helps get hydration to your skin and it makes your complexion even more dewy and beautiful. If you're going to eat B vitamins you can get them in bananas and rice.

Selenium – This mineral is attributed as one of the best for preventing skin cancer. Even if you have skin cancer it's been found to reduce some of your risks. And if you have trouble with burning? Selenium will help reduce the risk. The best place to find this mineral is in broccoli, cabbage, spinach, pinto beans and rice.

Copper – This one is great for elastin. That's what helps keep your skin smooth and young looking without all those wrinkles, lines, roughness and of course photo damage. You'll find it in legumes, spinach, kale, Swiss chard and mustard greens.

Zinc - Finally, if you have acne you want to try out zinc as your first method of curing it because a lack of zinc can actually cause acne. That's because it reduces your level of oils. If you want to get zinc you'll find it primarily in meats and poultry rather than fruit and vegetables.

You've probably heard this one before too but it's extremely important. Water is what hydrates your entire body and that goes for your skin as well. If you're not getting enough (and trust me I never used to get enough) your skin starts to suffer. The problem is your body takes the liquid that you do have and uses it for the most essential functions. Unfortunately for you, your skin quality is not considered one of those 'essential functions.'

So, if you don't drink enough water to take care of everything else that needs to be done your skin doesn't get any and that results in drying skin. Drying skin results in wrinkles. What that means is you get more problems with wrinkles just because you're not getting enough water in your diet and your skin cells aren't able to reproduce fast enough to keep your skin healthy.

By just drinking more water each day you improve the health of your skin and you start to look healthier and younger. This is because enough water is also going to give you a better glow to your skin and help you really *feel* younger too. The best thing to do is drink as much water as you can each day but that's not always easy for everyone to measure. I know that I never felt that thirsty but I was definitely dehydrated.

The best thing you can do is force yourself to drink water throughout the day. Instead of just deciding to drink when you're thirsty make sure that you actively drink when you're not. Take a gallon jug of water and make sure you drink at least that much water each day. It's going to help your skin (and the rest of your body) even more than you can imagine. Because if your skin is dehydrated then chances are you have some other organs in the body that are too. One gallon of water a day will help improve your overall health as well as your looks (which was a bonus for me).

Chapter 2: Too Much Vitamin D?

You may be one of those people who loves getting a great tan and adores sitting out in the sun all day when it's nice outside but there's one important thing you need to know: The sun is not your friend. In fact, when you're trying to get your skin looking great the sun is your absolute worst enemy. The reason? It counteracts everything you're trying to do to improve your health and makes your skin look worse than ever.

The sun will give you a tan, which is why most people like to go outside in it during the warm months. Unfortunately, it will also give you sunburn, wrinkles, dark spots and cancer. All of these make you look prematurely older than you actually are and the effects can actually be extremely dangerous as well.

I was never one of those people that sat out in the sun trying to get a tan all the time. I would go out occasionally but mostly it was just to get from one area to the other. My problem was that I never wore sunscreen. And when I say never? I mean absolutely *never*. I can count the number of times that I put sunscreen on in my entire life before I started trying to get my skin to look great and that would be two. In my entire life.

Because I don't have pale skin I assumed that I would never have a problem. I didn't burn at all and only had a slight tan after spending any amount of time outside. So I assumed that I didn't have to worry. Boy was I wrong. I actually have to worry even more because darker skin makes it harder to tell when damage is occurring. By wearing sunscreen, even when I'm not going to be outside very long, I can reduce the risk of damage of all types.

If you put sunscreen on before you go outside you'll be able to cut down dramatically on your risk of everything we mentioned from wrinkles and dark spots to sunburns and cancer. So just reducing your exposure to the sun is going to help you look much younger.

Chapter 3: How to Stop Worrying and Start Looking Younger

If you're anything like me then your first thought when you saw this chapter title was probably 'easier said than done.' Keeping your stress levels down is extremely important because stress causes you to breakout, it causes fine lines, and dehydration of the skin. If you already have rosacea or psoriasis it can even increase the problems you have with them.

So on top of everything that you probably know about stress and what it can do to your body you may also start looking older because you're worried more frequently. Unfortunately, as you start getting older you start stressing out even more as a matter of course. This makes it really difficult to cut down on since there never seems to be an end in sight.

If you can find a way to cut your stress levels however, you'll find that you actually feel better all-around as well as being able to make your skin look younger. I probably sound like an advertisement but it's absolutely true that cutting down on stress seemed to make a huge difference in my life. Like I said I had never had a big problem with acne as a child but when I got older it seemed I had acne all the time. That cut down drastically when I cut some stress out of my life.

The best things you can do for stress are to get rid of people that are just too toxic (the ones that are constantly making you feel bad about yourself) and to figure out a relaxation technique. For me it was reading. Whenever I feel like everything is just too overwhelming I take a few minutes to read a good book and it helps me get rid of the stress. Some people really like yoga or exercise for things like this so figure out what your best method of stress release is and go for it.

Chapter 4: How to Naturally Let Your Skin Repair Itself

Sleep rehydrates your skin and helps it to repair itself. When you're sleeping is when those cuts and scrapes start to heal up, it's when your muscles repair themselves from workouts and it's when your skin starts to recover from the sun, the wind, the cold, the heat and the dehydration. If you don't get enough sleep then all of these things just don't happen the way that they're supposed to so you end up with problems.

The average adult is supposed to get about 8 hours of sleep each night. Now I know for me this was nearly impossible for the longest time and I just finally had to put my foot down and say 'no, I'm not going to stay up until all hours of the night no matter what still needs to be done.' So I ended up getting ready for bed earlier every night and I felt much better. My skin started to look better too. The right amount of sleep gets rid of bags under your eyes and it helps your skin take on that dewy look that's so synonymous with healthy skin.

Chapter 5: What to Avoid

Have you seen some of the products that are available at the store for your skin? I definitely have. As I mentioned I tried a lot of those and I was surprised at how much they didn't work. Many of them have been out for years and have great reviews and yet they still didn't do anything for me. Well, maybe that's not fair. They did help me a little bit but they didn't seem to do nearly enough. (Compared to everything I got when I switched to natural methods they didn't do hardly anything.)

Unnatural products will generally have at least a few great ingredients in them. For example, they might have a lot of Vitamin C, which is great for your skin. But then they usually contain a lot of chemicals, additives and other 'extra stuff' that counteracts the benefits. Some of these will dry out your skin or they'll make you break out or they might just make you sick (which is also unhealthy for your skin).

Are there some products that you can buy in the store that are good for your skin? Yes, there are. I'm not going to tell you which products are going to work for you because I have no idea what the specific needs of your skin are. What I can tell you is all-natural and organic products are the best choice if you're going to buy anything in a store. Read through the ingredients list and if any of the ingredients aren't found in nature you don't want it.

There are a ton of all-natural beauty products that are good for your skin and these are available in everything you could possibly need. In fact, everything from body wash, cleansers and scrubs to eye shadow, mascara and lipstick are available in all-natural versions. I will admit that these brands are going to cost you a little more money but they're going to make it easier to get your skin healthy.

Chapter 6: Natural Skin Remedies to Use

Like I said, all natural products are the way to go. But you don't have to buy them at the store to get the benefits. You don't even need a lot of ingredients (whereas most store products will have a lot of different products mixed together). In fact, there are a lot of things that grow in nature that you can just apply to your skin and you'll get benefits. You don't have to mix them with anything at all, which makes it really easy to use them.

There are a ton of natural ingredients that you can use so I'm going to just list them first and then I'll tell you a little more about the ones that I use.

- Aloe Vera
- Calendula
- Cocoa Butter
- Cranberries
- Chamomile
- Coconut Oil
- Goji Berry
- Grape Seed Oil
- Green Tea
- Jojoba Oil
- Lavender
- Olive Oil
- Shea Butter
- Spearmint
- Sunflower Oil
- Zinc Oxide
- Vitamin C
- Tea Tree Oil

Personally, I've used a few of these and some of them I still do. For example, I still use olive oil on my skin because it helps to soothe my skin (it acts almost like a massage oil) and it also cuts down on pollution damage because it tones and firms up your skin as soon as you apply it; definitely awesome.

I've also used Shea butter on my own skin but I have to say I wasn't a fan. Not that it didn't work. The Shea butter that I used actually worked really well. It slows down aging in your skin and it also helps you get much more elasticity. The only problem I had with it was the smell. It doesn't smell bad (and you can get all different scents) but it's definitely not the same as other lotions.

The lotion that I love best is cocoa butter. I love the smell of this one (which is one of the reasons I chose it over Shea butter). I also love the way it restores the skin and gets rid of wrinkles. It has a lot of Vitamin E in it which means it gives you more moisturizing benefits at the same time as making your skin soft.

If you apply any of these to your skin you'll get benefits. Of course, those benefits will vary based on how often you use the product and when you're using it. Your skin actually absorbs earlier in the day or late at night so if you use these right when you get up or when you go to bed you'll see benefits a lot faster. Try out a few of them and see which work best for you. Some are better for removing wrinkles while others are best for smoothing out your skin or soothing irritation.

Chapter 7: The Game Plan

My plan is actually pretty simple. Like I said I've already gone through and tried out a lot of different fruits and vegetables as well as different products for my skin so I have pretty much figured out what I need to do. Plus, I work from home so I have a little more flexibility about how my day goes, when I eat and what I do overall.

This exact schedule may not work for you but try to stick close to it. It's actually proven to be really great for me and helps me feel better throughout the day. Maybe you don't have to get up as early as I do but try to take a few minutes for yourself every morning, drink plenty of water, eat breakfast and take breaks, plus eat snacks. All of these things will help you feel relaxed throughout the day and they're going to improve your skin a lot. So here's my schedule, see if you can make it (or something similar) work for you.

7:00am Wakeup- At this point in the day I like to take a few minutes to just relax. I'm awake but I generally don't actually get out of bed for another ten to fifteen minutes just so I can enjoy the quiet of the morning. From there I usually spend a little time getting through things like, putting another load of laundry in or skimming through my email. I also drink two glasses of water because drinking water about half an hour before you eat will help you feel less hungry so you eat less (which is important to overall health), plus it helps hydrate your body.

7:30am Eat Breakfast- I'm not a big breakfast person so my breakfast consists of a piece of fruit like an orange or a banana. If I'm really hungry in the morning I'll have a banana and some toast with peanut butter. It tastes really good so I don't actually feel like I'm eating healthy even though I am. If you need more calories in the morning consider oatmeal with apples or you can try my toast with peanut butter and bananas.

8:00am Get Ready for the Day- This is when I really get into my skin routine. I start out the same as everyone else with a shower and brushing my teeth, but after that I take some time to nourish my skin. This is when I use my cocoa butter which also helps me wake up a little more. I actually have a cocoa butter scrub which I use in the shower and a lotion that I use when I get out so I can get rid of dead skin cells and help regenerate the good ones.

8:30am Off to Work- By this time I'm done with my morning routine and I'm ready to work. It usually goes pretty smoothly for a while before I start to get a little anxious. That's when I know that it's time to take a break so I don't end up too stressed.

10:00am Break Time- By taking frequent breaks I'm able to relax and I never actually fall into the pit of 'too much stress.' So I take about 15-20 minutes just to read a little before I go back to work. During this entire time I'm drinking more water and keeping an eye on my intake. If I'm hungry I might have a few grapes or nuts.

12:30pm Lunch Time- Lunch usually consists of something light. I make myself eat some protein (since I'm really not a meat person) but it's usually far outweighed by the fruits. In fact, one of my favorite things to eat for lunch is fruit salad which I make by myself because I like everything to be completely natural rather than the processed stuff you get from a can. Once again, I'm drinking more water half an hour before and during my meal as well. For some protein I might eat some yogurt with granola or seeds in it or maybe some beans if I decide to opt for a regular salad instead.

2:00pm Break Time- Once again it's time to take a break. That means reducing stress by relaxing with my book, drinking more water and having a little more fruit as a snack. When I get back to work I feel less stress and I'm ready to get some more work done.

5:00pm Dinner Time- So now it's time for dinner. Unlike the rest of my day, at this point my entire family is there and that means eating a little more substantial food. My family doesn't like the rather light meals I eat the rest of the day so at dinner I try to make something that's a little heavier. We might have some chicken or steak with some type of fruit and a vegetable. It's enough food for everyone but it's still not too heavy where it's going to cause damage to my skin.

10:00pm Bed- At this point my day is over. I take a few minutes to relax by myself and I also follow up my skin routine. If I wore makeup that day (I don't always) I make sure to clean it off with some makeup remover cloths that are all-natural. I also have a brush I use to clean dirt and dead skin cells off my face at night. I follow that up with my moisturizer again and head to bed so I can get enough sleep to be up and ready in the morning for another day.

As I said you don't need to follow this program. What you should do is follow some of the basic ideas in it.

1. First thing in the morning relax on your own and drink plenty of water.
2. Eat a healthy breakfast of fruit (or fruit with some protein).
3. Get ready for your day by following your moisturizing, cleansing routine for your face.
4. Keep drinking water throughout the day.
5. Take a break partway through the morning even if you can't walk away for long.
6. Make sure your break consists of some method to relieve stress and a small snack of some fruit, nuts, seeds or some vegetables like carrot sticks or celery.
7. Lunch should consist of more fruit and some protein. If you're a big eater you might want a sandwich or you might eat leftovers. That's fine just try to make sure you don't feel stuffed when you're done (a sign you overate) and that you're still getting fruit which balances out some of the heavier food.
8. Take a break partway through the afternoon even if you can't walk away for long.
9. Once again make sure your break has a stress reliever and a small snack (if you're hungry).
10. You should still be drinking plenty of water throughout the day.
11. At dinner eat a little bit heartier. You might want a heavier protein and you'll want to include fruit and vegetables in your meal if at all possible.

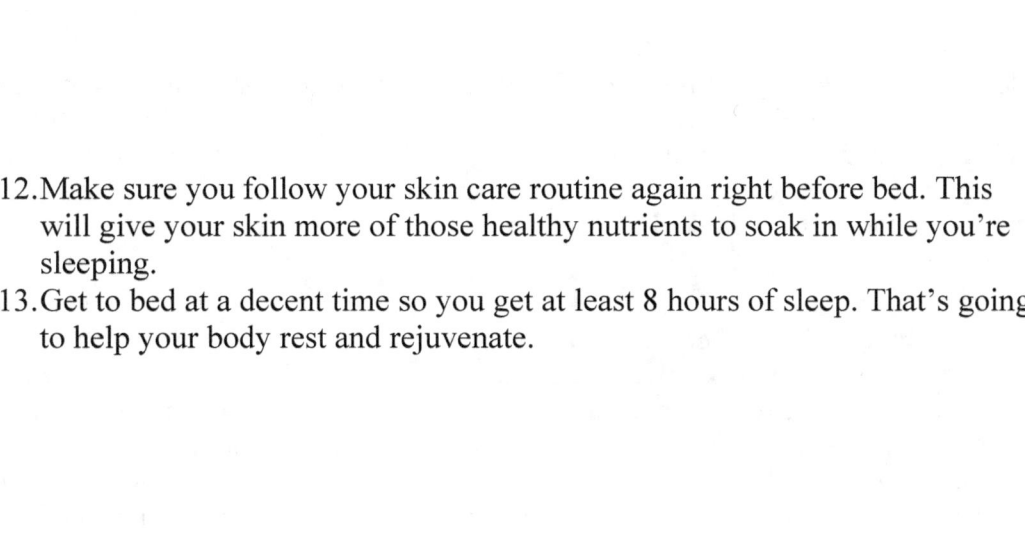

12. Make sure you follow your skin care routine again right before bed. This will give your skin more of those healthy nutrients to soak in while you're sleeping.
13. Get to bed at a decent time so you get at least 8 hours of sleep. That's going to help your body rest and rejuvenate.

Conclusion

You know that feeling when you're 15 and you get mistaken for being 20? You know how you get all excited and think it's so great that you look older? Well try being older and getting mistaken for a teenager. It's a way better feeling and that's a feeling I actually get to experience often. My skin care routine has actually made it possible for me to look like I'm 18 again and that's an awesome feeling.

If you want to look younger then go for it. You don't have to follow my routine exactly or even close to exactly. Instead, look for products that work best for you (for example, I have really oily skin so the cocoa butter helps to reduce that while others might like different products better so they get benefits for dry skin or combination skin). The basic points are important, more sleep, more water, healthy food, vitamins and minerals, breaks and all natural products. You'll feel better and you'll look younger and isn't that the most important part?